It Starts with Good Food:
Amazing Recip
Weight and

Henry Brooke

Table of Contents

Introduction

I want to thank you for downloading this book and taking the first step on your weight loss journey. Following the plan outlined in this book is a great way for you to reset your body and get on the right track to losing weight. Whether you want to get your body prepared for another diet plan that you want to be on for the long term or you are just ready to lose some weight and start eating right, this book will help you get there.

- Henry Brooke

Chapter 1: Tenants of the plan

Many different weight loss plans are available for you to choose from in order to lose some of the weight that is hanging on to your body. People are often confused about which diet they should choose just because so many of them are different from each other, some safe and some not, but they all promise to make a difference in your weight and whole life.

This is a program mirrored off of the Whole 30 diet plan that was started in 2009 and has helped many people get the results that they want when it comes to weight loss. On this diet plan, you will be able to eat some real food instead of having to eat prepackaged meals that are sent to you and have no flavor. You are allowed to eat the good fats that come from seeds, nuts, and oils, you are allowed to eat fruits and vegetables as well as eggs, seafood, and meat. You are told to eat foods that have either only a few ingredients in them, all of the ingredients can be pronounced, or foods that do not have any ingredients in them at all to start with since they are unprocessed. Unlike the whole 30 plan we believe that this can be an endeavor that lasts longer than 30 days and believe that paleo-ified snacks are ok with a longer term perspective.

So to summarize this point, some of the foods that you are allowed to eat would include things like:

- Meats—make sure they are lean meats with lots of protein. It is ok to have some more fatty meats on occasion, but these can be hard on your heart.
- Seafood—these have all of the great omega 3s that your body needs to stay healthy and happy with lots of protein.
- Eggs—you can also get a lot of protein as well as the B vitamins that your body needs from the eggs you eat.
- Vegetables—load up on all the vegetables you would like to eat with this diet.
- A few fruits—fruits are not the enemy here, but you do need to be careful. It is important that you just east some of the nutrition but be wary about the added sugar and carbs that come with them.
- Good fats—these would be the fats from products such as seeds, nuts, oils, and the fruits that you choose.

The more important thing on this diet is the foods that you should avoid. For a whole 30 days, you will need to omit the foods that are below. These are important because they are going to help with reducing the inflammation that you are feeling while revving up your metabolism and giving you a better quality of life. Some of the things that you will need to avoid on this diet include:

- Sugar—you should never eat any sugar, whether it is real or artificial. This includes syrup, coconut sugar, equal or anything else like this.
- Alcohol you should not use alcohol in any form, even if you wanted to use it for cooking. Avoid tobacco products as well.
- Grains—just like with the paleo diet, you will want to make sure that you are not eating grains. This would include any of the gluten free grains as well as your traditional grains such as bulgur, millet, corn, rice, barley, rye, and wheat.
- Legumes—these would include beans of all kinds as well as all soy forms and even peanut butter.
- Dairy—dairy of any kind is not allowed on this diet plan. This would include things such as cream cheese, goats or cow's milk, sour cream, and yogurt.
- Sulfites, MSG, or carrageenan—if you see these ingredients on any labels you are choosing, avoid them.

In addition to the foods that you are avoiding, you need to be able to get rid of the scale, at least for a month. While you are doing this program, you will need to just focus on eating the right foods and being healthy. Do not worry about the number on the scale or the measurements of your body during this time.

There are also a few foods that are exceptions to the rules put above. These foods can be included into the diet just like the allowed foods listed above. Some of the exceptions include:

- Ghee or clarified butter—this is the only form of dairy that you can have on the program.
- Fruit juice—this is the only sweetener that you can use on this program and apple and orange juice work well.
- Some legumes-you are allowed to have some of the legumes that are normally thought of as vegetables. These would include options such as snow peas, snap peas, and green beans.

- Vinegar—most of the forms of vinegar, such as rice, red wine, apple cider, balsamic, and white, are allowed on the program.
- Salt—you can have some salt on the diet, just use it carefully because you do not want to increase your blood pressure too much.

So now that you know what you can eat, you are probably curious about why you should go about doing it. The diet is not that complicated and can be found in other low carb diets that are on the market. You will still need to exercise and go about your daily business, but you just need to make smarter decisions about the foods that you are eating. It might be tough getting through some of those ravings in the beginning, but a little bit of hard work and it will yield amazing results.

This program is only going to take you 30 days, but you have to remain completely true to it. You cannot cheat, have special occasions, or slip up on the diet because that is going to ruin the results that you are getting out of it. It can be a bit tough in the beginning, but with some dedication and following the rules, you will be amazed at how much weight you can lose.

Chapter 2: Amazing Breakfasts

Sweet Potatoes and Fried Eggs

½ an onion
2 sausages
1 pepper, bell
1 Tbsp. oil, coconut
1 sweet potato
4 eggs
Pepper

Take out a skillet and heat up a little bit of coconut oil on your stove. Once the oil has had time to heat up, you can add in the onions with the sweet potatoes. Let these two ingredients sauté for 5 minutes and then add your sausage in. Continue the cooking process until your sausage is turning brown and the sweet potatoes begin to soften. Finally add a little water and the bell peppers before covering the mixture up and allowing everything to cook for another 15 minutes. While the vegetables are all cooking, you can bring out another pan and fry up the eggs with the remaining oil until cooked all the way through. Mix together the hash brown and eggs before placing on a plate. Add some pepper for seasoning and enjoy.

Carrot and Banana Muffins

2 tsp. baking soda
Cinnamon
3 eggs
Apple cider vinegar
¾ c. walnuts
2 c. almond flour
Salt
1 c. dates, pitted
3 bananas
¼ c. oil, coconut
1 ½ c. carrots

To start this recipe you can turn on the oven so it can heat up to 350 degrees. Next, you can take out a bowl and combine the salt, flour, cinnamon, and baking soda. Set this bowl aside while you continue. Taking out a blender, combine the vinegar, bananas, oil, eggs, and dates and then add this mixture in with the dry ingredients. Fold the carrots and the nuts into the mixture and then spoon it all into your muffin tins. After the tins are full, you can place them in the oven and allow the muffins to bake for 25 minutes. When the muffins are done cooking, you can take them from the oven and allow them some time to cool and then enjoy.

Pancakes

1 Tbsp. coconut flour
1 c. almond flour
2 eggs
Salt
Coconut oil
½ c. unsweetened applesauce
¼ tsp. nutmeg
¼ c. water
Berries

Taking out a bowl, combine the almond flour, applesauce, coconut flour, eggs, water, nutmeg, and salt. You will want to make sure that everything is mixed well together before continuing. Next you can take out a skillet and place it and some coconut oil on the stove. When the skillet is warmed up, take about ¼ of your batter and drop it on the skillet. Once the edges start to bubble a little, you can flip your pancake over and allow the other side to cook. Repeat this process so that you use up the batter. When all of the pancakes are done you can top on fresh berries and enjoy.

Tapioca Crepes

1 c. water
1 c. flour, tapioca flour
Pinch salt
1 egg
Berries for topping.

To begin this recipe, you can bring out a bowl and combine together the tapioca flour, water, egg, and salt, making sure to mix them all together well. Next, heat up et on the stove and wait for it to get warm. Once the skillet is warm, pour about 1/3 of the mixture into the skillet. Tilt the skillet all around so the mixture is the thickness that you want. You will want to cook the crepe for about 2 minutes on both sides before taking off the heat and putting on a plate. Place the berries or other toppings that you want on the crepes and enjoy!

Summer Frittata

1 diced zucchini
1 ½ Tbsp. olive oil
½ diced bell pepper, red
½ diced red onion
½ tsp. salt
1 Tbsp. thyme
¼ tsp. pepper
1 tomato
2 minced cloves of garlic
9 eggs

For this recipe, you can heat up the coconut oil in a skillet. Once it has a chance to heat up, you can add in the garlic, a little pepper and salt, the thyme, onion, pepper, and zucchini to the skillet. Cover the skillet up and let the vegetables cook for about 5 minutes so that they can become tender. After this time, you can stir the tomato in and let it cook for another 5 minutes so the liquid can evaporate. While that is cooking up, you can bring out a bowl and combine the eggs with the rest of the pepper and salt, making sure to whisk until it becomes frothy. When the vegetables are ready, pour your eggs on top of them before covering, reducing the heat, and continue cooking for another 15 minutes. Turn the broiler on next and let it heat up to a low setting. The frittata will need to be placed into the broiler for about 3 minutes to set before enjoying.

Western Omelet

1 tsp. coconut oil
4 eggs
1 diced bell pepper
½ diced yellow onion
1 diced tomato
¼ lbs. cooked ham
1 c. spinach
Salt
Pepper

Take the vegetables and wash them off before chopping them into smaller pieces and setting aside. Next, bring out a bowl and crack the eggs in it before beating them well and setting aside as well. Place the coconut oil on a skillet and let it heat up before pouring half of your egg mixture onto the bottom of your skillet. When it has had some time to set, you can scrape off the edges and tip around the pan so the rest of the egg can get cooked. Now you can take the ham and the vegetables and place it on half of the omelet. Continue cooking for a few more minutes so the egg can finish setting. Using your spatula, fold the egg in half and cook for two more minutes. Repeat these steps with the rest of the ingredients to get another omelet and then enjoy!

Berry Zucchini Muffins

½ c. coconut flour
1 c. almond flour
2 tsp. baking soda
½ c. tapioca flour
1 tsp. salt
1 Tbsp. allspice
1 Tbsp. cinnamon
1 c. pitted dates
3 eggs
3 bananas
1 tsp. vinegar, apple cider
5 oz. frozen berries
¼ c. coconut oil
¾ c. almonds
¾ c. zucchini

Give your berries some time to thaw out before beginning this recipe. While the berries are thawing out, you can turn on the oven and let it warm up to 350 degrees. Next, take out a bowl and combine together the allspice, cinnamon, salt, baking soda, tapioca flour, coconut flour, and the almond flour. Bring out your food processor and combine together the oil, vinegar, eggs, bananas, and dates before transferring to another bowl and stirring to combine with the other ingredients. Slowly fold in the almonds, zucchini, and berries next before spooning this mixture into your muffin tin and placing into the oven. Allow the muffins to bake for about 20 minutes or until they are completely done.

Chapter 3: Mouth Watering Lunches

Taco Salad

Garlic salt
Oregano
Cumin
1 lb. ground beef
¾ c. water
Salt
2 Tbsp. powder, chili
1 tomato
3 romaine hearts
½ yellow onion
1 c. black olives
1 avocado
1 can salsa
Cilantro

Take out a skillet and let it heat up over the stove. Once the skillet is warm you can add in the beef and onion and let them both cook for 10 minute so that the meat has time to brown up. After the beef is browned you can add in the chili powder, cumin, salt, oregano, garlic salt, and water and let everything simmer for an additional 5 minutes. Next you can take the romaine lettuce and wash it off before dividing it between two serving plates. Top your lettuce with the meat mixture, black olives, salsa, avocado, and cilantro before serving.

Salad with Beef Stir Fry

2 tsp. coconut oil
2 peppers, bell
1 ½ lbs. beef steak tips
1 Tbsp. coconut aminos
Peapods
2 heads of lettuce
Salt
½ sweet onion
Olive oil
Pepper
Balsamic vinegar

For this recipe, you can take out a skillet and let it heat up on the oven and then add on the coconut oil. After the skillet has warmed up, you can add in the onions and allow them time to sauté so they can become soft. Turn the heat up a little and then add the beef and coconut aminos, allowing them to cook until the beef is about done. At this time you should add the bell peppers and the peas into the mixture. Season this whole mixture with the pepper and the salt before serving on top of your lettuce heads. Add a little bit of balsamic vinegar if you would like for taste.

Paleo Chili

6 cloves of garlic
1 green pepper, bell
2 lbs. beef
Pepper
2 Tbsp. oil, olive
1 ½ Tbsp. chili powder
1 can tomatoes, diced
3 Tbsp. cumin

This recipe will start out by forming the beef into patties. Heat a little of the oil into a soup pot before adding the black pepper into it. Next, take the bell peppers and sauté them in the oil in the soup pot for 7 minutes before taking the pot from the heat. Stir the garlic next and then set the pot aside for a few minutes. Turn your grill on before placing the beef patties on it and allowing the meat to cook so they become medium rare. At this time, you can turn back on the heat and place the soup pot back on the stove before adding the garlic, oil, and pepper into the pot, making sure to break up the patties so they are small pieces before adding. Finally, add the tomatoes to the mixture, making sure to mash them up well before adding some water so that the ingredients become covered. Allow the whole chili to simmer for a minimum of two hours and then enjoy.

Grilled Veggies and Shrimp on a Stick

Juice from 1 lime
¾ lb. shrimp
1 sliced zucchini
Pepper
1 sliced summer squash, yellow
1 sliced bell pepper, red
1 sliced bell pepper, green
3 Tbsp. olive oil
4 minced garlic gloves, skewers

To start this recipe, you can take your shrimp and peel it before placing into a bowl. Add the pepper and the lime juice to the bowl and let it all set to the side for about five minutes. While the shrimp is soaking, you can take your vegetables and wash and chop them up. Turn on the grill at this time so that it has time to warm up. Add your garlic, olive oil, and vegetables to the bowl with the shrimp and toss to combine. Place the shrimp and the veggies onto the skewers and then place on the grill to cook. After everything is well cooked, you can take off the grill and enjoy.

Chicken Fajitas

3 minced garlic cloves
1 tsp. oregano
1 tsp. cumin
1 tsp. chili powder
1 lb. chicken breast
1 tsp. salt
1 Tbsp. coconut oil
2 sliced bell peppers, red
½ sliced red onion
Juice from 1 lemon
Juice from 1 lime
Guacamole
2 heads of lettuce
1 jar salsa

Bring out a bowl and combine together the salt, chili powder, oregano, cumin, and garlic together. Toss the chicken in with this mixture so that it can become coated on all sides and then set aside. Next, heat up a sauté pan with the coconut oil. When it is warmed up, you can place the onion inside the onion for about 3 minutes before adding in the chicken and let it all cook for another 10 minutes so that the chicken is cooked through. Right before the chicken finishes, you can add in the lime juice, lemon juice, and red peppers. Cook everything for another 3 minutes. Serve everything over the lettuce and top with some salsa and guacamole before enjoying.

Chicken Thai Wraps

1 lb. chicken breasts
4 cabbage leaves
12 lettuce leaves
1 c. chopped raw broccoli
3 sliced green onions
1 shredded carrot
Cilantro
Thai Sauce
¼ c. water
¼ c. almond butter
2 Tbsp. lime juice
2 Tbsp. coconut aminos
2 minced garlic cloves

Start this recipe by grilling up the chicken until it is completely cooked and then dice into cubes. Next, take the leaves of lettuce and spread them onto a plate. Fill the lettuce leaves with cilantro, green onions, carrots, cabbage, broccoli, and chicken. Next, take all of the ingredients for the Thai sauce and combine them together in a bowl. Drizzle this sauce over the rest of the ingredients and then enjoy!

Portobello Sandwich

¼ c. almond butter
4 mushroom caps
4 slices bacon
Handful spinach
1 sliced tomato
¼ sliced yellow onion
1 sliced avocado

Take each of your mushroom caps and spread out some of the almond butter on the bottom of each way. Next, take the bacon and vegetables and layer them over 2 of the mushroom caps. Top with the rest of the Portobello caps before enjoying

Chapter 4: Delicious Dinners

Paleo Pizza

2 eggs
3 Tbsp. butter, almond
1 c. flour, almond
Salt
4 mushrooms
3 tsp. oil, olive
½ c. yellow onion
2 cloves of garlic
1 Italian sausage
1 pepper, red
Fennel seed
½ c. cherry tomatoes
Oregano
½ c. sauce, marinara sauce

For this recipe you will need to turn the oven up so it reaches 350 degrees. While the oven is heating up, you can take out a bowl and mix together the almond flour, almond butter, eggs, and salt. Before placing this mixture into the baking dish, you can spread out some olive oil onto the bottom. Place the mixture into your oven and allow it time to bake, around 10 minutes. During the cooking process, you can take out a skillet and cook together the onions, mushrooms, and sausage and heat it up in order to cook the sausage. Set this aside and then add the garlic and red pepper to your skillet, making sure to sauté the vegetables for around 3 minutes. When the crust is done, you can add in both the mixtures that you just did into it and sprinkle with the spices. Place this whole dish in the oven and allow another 20 minutes to cook. When the pizza is done, you can take it out of the oven and top with your tomatoes before enjoying.

Tasty Spaghetti

1 lb. ground beef
1 Tbsp. oil, olive
24 oz. noodles, kelp
2 cloves of garlic
15 oz. sauce, marinara

To start this recipe, you can heat up your skillet and add in some olive oil. When the olive oil has heated up, you can add in the garlic and the meat and allow them to cook for a few minutes, making sure the meat has been completely heated up before continuing. Next, add in the noodles along with the marinara sauce and let everything cook to a simmer. When it is all heated up, take off the stove and enjoy.

Paleo Burgers

Salt
Pepper
1 lb. ground beef
Coconut oil

This easy recipe will start by taking out a bowl and mixing together the salt and pepper with the meat. Once everything is properly mixed together, you can take it and form 4 patties that are about even. Next, take out a skillet and warm it up on the oven and then add in the coconut oil. Cook the patties of beef on the skillet until they reach your desired doneness. Make sure to serve the burgers along with some healthy toppings.

Sloppy Joes

1 onion
2 Tbsp. olive oil
1 lb. ground beef
1 green pepper
1 can sauce, tomato
2 cloves of garlic
Chili powder
Cumin

To start this recipe you can take a skillet and heat it up while adding in the oil. After the oil is heated up, you can add in the green pepper, onion, and garlic and allow these vegetables to sauté for at least 10 minutes. You will want them to become tender before continuing. Once the vegetables are tender, you can add in your beef and continuing cooking so the beef starts to become brown, which will take another 10 minutes. Finally, add in the tomato sauce, cumin, and chili powder to this mixture. When everything is combined, you can take it off the heat before serving.

Macadamia Halibut

¾ c. chopped Macadamia nuts
1 egg
1 tsp. olive oil
2 tsp. water
1 Tbsp. chopped parsley
¼ tsp. salt
1 lb. halibut fillets
¼ tsp. pepper
1 sliced orange
Zest from half an orange

Start this recipe by turning on the oven and letting it warm up to 350 degrees. Next, take out a skillet and toast up the Macadamia nuts so they turn a little brown. Allow them to cool down so that you can chop them into smaller pieces. Take out a baking dish and grease it up with some olive oil and set aside. Bringing out a bowl, you can beat together the water and the egg before setting aside. Add the orange zest, nuts, pepper, salt, and parsley in another bowl. Now you can take the halibut fillet into the egg mixture, making sure to coat each side, before pressing into your nut mixture. Make sure it is completely coated. Place your fillets into the prepared pan and let it bake in the oven for about 15 minutes. Serve the fish with the orange slices and then serve right away.

Lime and Dill Crab

2 Dungeness crabs
1 tsp. paprika
Juice from 1 lime
2 tsp. chopped dill

To start this recipe, you can take out a pot full of water and heat it up so that the water starts to boil. Once the water starts boiling, drop the crabs in and let them cook for about 8 minutes. After that time, you can take the crabs out of the water and put them under some cold water so they become easy to handle. When the crab has cooled down, crack the shells and take the meat out before drizzling on the dill, paprika, and lime juice. Serve this dish with some lime wedges and enjoy.

Vegetable and Turkey Meatballs

2 carrots
1 lb. ground chicken
1 bell pepper, green
5 mushrooms
Handful parsley
1 garlic clove
½ yellow onion
2 tsp. garlic salt
½ tsp. pepper
2 Tbsp. Italian seasoning

Preheat the oven so that it can warm up to 350 degrees. While the oven is heating up, you can combine together the seasonings, garlic, onion, mushrooms, bell pepper, and carrots to your food processor. Let them blend so they become well chopped up. Empty these ingredients into a bowl before adding the ground chicken and mixing everything together well. When the ingredients are mixed, you can form them into meatballs before placing onto a baking sheet and placing into the oven. Allow the meatballs to bake for 25 minutes before serving.

Meat Loaf

1 tsp. salt
¼ tsp. sage
1 tsp. dry mustard
1 tsp. garlic salt
½ tsp. pepper
1 tsp. chili powder, chipotle
1 chopped yellow onion
4 garlic cloves
1 c. chopped red cabbage
½ tsp. hot pepper sauce
2 tbsp. water
1 beaten egg
1/3 c. almond meal
½ c. barbecue sauce
1 ½ lbs. ground beef

Start this recipe by preheating the oven so that it can warm up to 350 degrees. Bring out a bowl and combine together all of the ingredients except the barbecue sauce and ground beef, making sure to mix well. When the ingredients are well blended, you can add in the beef and combine using a fork. Place this mixture in a loaf pan and pour the barbecue sauce all over the meatloaf. Place the loaf pan into the oven and let it bake for about 75 minutes. At this time, you can take out of the oven and allow it to set for about 5 minutes before slicing and serving.

Pot Roast

2 lb. pot roast, beef
2 Tbsp. beef tallow
2 sliced yellow onion
3 carrots
2 celery stalks
1 bay leaf
½ tsp. pepper
1 Tbsp. thyme
Salt
½ tsp. oregano
3 c. water

To begin this recipe, bring out a bowl and mix together the salt, oregano, thyme, and pepper. Use this mixture to rub all over the roast. Take out a skillet next and heat it up on the stove before placing some of the beef tallow when it is hot. Place the roast in the skillet and cook it on each side for a few minutes in order to sear it on each side before setting aside for later. While the roast is cooking, you can prepare and wash the vegetables. Bring out your crock pot and place the roast inside before adding the water, bay leaf, and vegetables. Cover the crock pot and cook on a high setting for about 6 hours. Serve when you are ready.

Pork Chops

¼ tsp. pepper
½ tsp. salt
¼ tsp. paprika
¼ tsp. thyme
¼ tsp. sage
1 Tbsp. lard
4 pork chops
1 sliced onion

Start this recipe by preheating your oven so that it can heat up to 425 degrees. While the oven is heating up, you can take out a bowl and mix together the thyme, sage, paprika, pepper, and salt. Use this mixture to season the pork chops. Take out a skillet and heat it up with the lard on the oven. When the skillet is warm, you can place the pork chops in the skillet and let them brown on each side. Place your cooked chops on some tin foil before layering with the onions, close the foil, and place it onto a baking sheet. Bake the pork chops in the oven for about 30 minutes or until completely cooked. Serve the pork chops right away after they are done cooking and enjoy!

Chapter 5: Craving Curing Snacks

Deviled Eggs with Guacamole

1 avocado
4 hard-boiled eggs
2 tsp. hot sauce
Salt
1 tsp. lemon juice
Pepper

To start this recipe, you will want to hard-boil your eggs using your favorite recipe. When that is done, you can peel them before cutting in half going length wise. Spoon out the yolks from the eggs into a bowl before mashing them together with the lemon juice, hot sauce, and avocado. Make sure to season with a little bit of pepper and salt for taste. Once the mixture is done, you can refill your eggs with it and then serve.

Peanut Butter and Jelly

4 Tbsp. almond butter
1 c. berries

For this recipe, you can bring out two bowls and divide up your berries between them. Once you are done with that, take the almond butter and divide it between the two bowls as well. Make sure to mix the ingredients together well before enjoying.

Plantains

Coconut oil or ghee
1 plantain
Salt
Chili powder

Melt a tablespoon of the oil into a skillet and let it heat up. Choose the plantain, getting one that is dull with some black patches. Cut off the end and then split up the plantain so it is in half before laying it into the prepared skillet. Cook for about 2 minutes before turning over and doing the same on the other side. Turn over two more times to cook for another 4 minutes. At this time, move to a plate and then dust on the chili powder and the salt all over before enjoying the plantains.

Grape Fruit Salad

2 Tbsp. chopped cashews
½ c. coconut flakes
2 grapefruits
½ minced shallot
1/3 c. mint leaves
1 Tbsp. minced shrimp
1/2 minced jalapeno
Juice from a lime
½ juiced orange
1 Tbsp. fish sauce

Heat up a pan on the stove. When it becomes hot, toss the cashews and coconut flakes inside. Let these toast for about 5 minutes and then take out of the pan to cool down before you continue. Over a bowl catch the juice of the grapefruit and then get the juice from the membranes. Section the fruit and then get rid of the membranes so that you just have the fruit. Place into the bowl. IN another bowl you can whisk the orange juice, fish sauce, lime juice, jalapeno, shrimp, shallot, and mint. Add in the grapefruit and then fold to combine. Sprinkle in the cashews and coconut and then fold again. Allow to set for 10 minutes to let it all mix together before you start to eat the snack.

Conclusion

Thank you for downloading this book!

I hope this book helps you jumpstart your journey to an amazing 30 days and beyond on the It starts with good food cookbook. It can be tough the first few days but I encourage you to stick with it. You'll be feeling better in no time. I wish you the best of luck and success 30 days and beyond!!

Finally, if you enjoyed this book, then I'd like to ask you for a favor, would you be kind enough to leave a review for this book on Amazon? It'd be greatly appreciated!

Thank you and good luck!

- Henry Brooke

Made in the USA
Monee, IL
19 May 2022

96696245R00017